# Hormone Reset Diet

## *Over 30 Hormone Reset Diet Recipes to Balanced Hormones, FAST Weight Loss, Lower Stress, Better Immune System, and Faster Metabolism*

# PS: I Owe You!

Thank you for stopping by.

My name is Antony and I am passionate about teaching people literally everything I know about different aspects of life. I am an author and a ghostwriter. I run a small ghostwriting company with slightly over 100 writers. My wife (Faith) and I manage the business along with several other members of the team (editors).

Nice to meet you!

I started publishing (at Fantonpublishers.com) because I'd love to impart the knowledge I gather every single day in my line of work (reading and editing over 10 ghostwritten books every single day). My ghostwriting company deals with literally every topic under the sun, which puts me at a very unique position to learn more in a month than I learnt in my 4 years as a Bachelor of Commerce, Accounting, student. I am constantly answering questions from my friends, relatives and even strangers on various topics that I come across every day at work.

After several years of helping people to achieve different goals (e.g. weight loss, making money online, human resources, management, investing, stress reduction, depression, budgeting, saving etc.) offline thanks to my 'street' as well as 'class' knowledge on different topics, I realized I could be of better help to the world by publishing what I learn. My books are a reflection of what I have been gathering over the years. That's why they are not just focused on one niche but every niche possible out there.

If you would love to be part of my lovely audience who want to change multiple aspects of their life, subscribe to our newsletter http://bit.ly/2fantonpubnewbooks or follow us on social media to receive notifications whenever we publish new books on any niche. You can also send me an email; I would love to hear from you!

**PS**: Valuable content is my bread and butter. And since I have lots of it to go around, I can share it freely (not everything is about money - **changing lives comes first!**)

*I promise; I am busy just as you are and won't spam (I hate spam too)!*

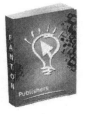

**Antony,**

**Website**: http://www.fantonpublishers.com/

**Email:** Support@fantonpublishers.com

**Twitter**: https://twitter.com/FantonPublisher

**Facebook Page**:
https://www.facebook.com/Fantonpublisher/

**Private Facebook Group For Readers:**
https://www.facebook.com/groups/FantonPublishers/

**Pinterest**: https://www.pinterest.com/fantonpublisher/

*Some of the best things in life are free, right?*

As a sign of good faith, I will start by giving out content that will help you to implement not only everything I teach in this book but in every other book I write. The content is about life transformation, presented in bit size pieces for easy implementation. I believe that without such a checklist, you are likely to have a hard time implementing anything in this book and any other thing you set out to do religiously and sticking to it for the long haul. It doesn't matter whether your goals relate to weight loss, relationships, personal finance, investing, personal development, improving communication in your family, your overall health, finances, improving your sex life, resolving issues in your relationship, fighting PMS successfully, investing, running a successful business, traveling etc. With a checklist like the one I will show you, you can bet that anything you do will seem a lot easier to implement until the end. This checklist will help you to start well and not lose steam along the way, until the very end. Therefore, even if you don't continue reading this book, at least read the one thing that will help you in every other aspect of your life.

Send me a message on <u>support@fantonpublishers.com</u> and I will send you my 5 Pillar Life Transformation Checklist.

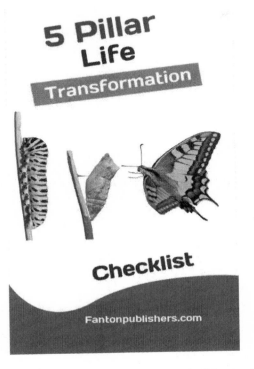

*Your life will never be the same again (if you implement what's in this book), I promise.*

# Introduction

Over 30 percent of the world's population is struggling with obesity. So what do you think is the problem? Is it that this population seems to eat too much of processed foods, which are high in empty calories or is it that our sedentary lifestyle is the reason behind the weight? Well, while this is all true, to some extent, this isn't really the root problem. That's why many of us who struggle with weight try one diet plan after another hoping to lose a few pounds and keep it off. While some of these diet plans actually help you lose weight, they don't help you keep it off because they don't handle the root cause of the problem. That's why you will probably gain all the weight you gained after a few weeks of being off the diet plan. So what is the problem? Well, I'd answer this with a single word; hormones.

As you will realize, lack of exercise and excessive calorie consumption are not really the reason why you often find it hard to lose weight and keep it off; hormonal imbalance is the reason. Your hormones are responsible for many of the body processes that take place so if something is wrong, you might end up accumulating belly fat even when you really don't see yourself consuming too many calories. Haven't you noticed that some skinny people tend to eat a lot more than you do yet they hardly gain all the weight?

If you often wonder what really makes you fat given the fact that you don't eat too many calories and probably engage in physical activities, your best solution to your weight problem is resetting your hormones to restore balance. And in so doing, you will not only lose weight but also derive many other benefits including improving your sex drive, feeling energetic and a lot more.

So how can you reset your hormones? Obviously, there's no "factory reset button" in the body so you need to learn how to do it correctly. One way of doing that is through diet and this book will help you to do just that.

You will learn what could be causing an imbalance in your hormones, the benefits of resetting your hormones and some recipes you can prepare to reset you hormones.

I hope you enjoy it!

# Table of Contents

# Different Hormones And How To Reset Them

Losing weight does not just entail changing your diet and exercising only. Sometimes, your hormones are haywire and this could be making it hard for you to lose weight and keep it off. Some hormones that can affect your weight loss goals include insulin, estrogen, cortisol and, leptin. The different hormones may require you to do different things to reset them. Let us look at this closely to help you understand more about hormone resetting.

You can reset your hormones by eliminating specific foods from your diet to bring your hormones back to balance.

## Sugar free diet

Sugar free diet resets insulin hormone.

Insulin is the hormone responsible for regulating the absorption of sugar (glucose) in the body cells i.e. it is the hormone, which usually tells the cells to start picking up glucose from the bloodstream. Besides that role, it is the hormone, which is responsible for energy storage in the body i.e. it actually signals the cells to start storing energy either as fat or as glycogen. Studies actually show a positive relationship between insulin levels and weight gain.

So how does that work?

Let's start from the beginning:

Whenever you eat any food, this is usually broken down into some basic nutrients (carbs are broken down into glucose, dietary fats into fatty acids and proteins into amino acids). These nutrients are then absorbed into the bloodstream. These are not yet available for the cells to use and it is only until insulin is produced that these nutrients are able to move from the bloodstream into fat cells and muscle cells for use or storage. This insulin is produced in the pancreas and as more nutrients are availed in the blood, more insulin is produced in order to trigger the cells to absorb/take up more of these nutrients for burning into energy or for storage. And as more of these nutrients are absorbed into the cells, insulin levels drop until all the nutrients have been absorbed after which insulin levels remain low but steady (this is known as the baseline level). The pancreas then "waits" until you eat again to release more insulin as more nutrients are availed in the blood.

When you take a diet high in calories (especially highly processed foods), the pancreas is prompted to release more insulin to facilitate in the absorption of the nutrients into the body cells for energy or storage. The high carb foods are responsible for causing the highest production of insulin after a meal. Keep in mind that insulin is also a fat storing hormone. So if you produce more insulin due to high calories in your bloodstream, this means that you will also be storing more calories as fat. This in itself makes it hard to burn body fat. And as you keep on producing insulin, the cells start losing their sensitivity to the insulin such that you will need more insulin to trigger the cells to take absorb these nutrients. If this goes on for a long time, this results to a condition referred to as hyperinsulinemia, a condition whereby insulin levels are high all the time; this is caused by insulin resistance, a precursor to diabetes.

The more insulin resistant you become, the more of unused nutrients that remain in your bloodstream. While some of this might be eliminated through urine, much of it is stored as fat in different parts of the body. Actually, insulin resistance comes with increased ability to store fat easily coupled with increased triglycerides, cholesterol and blood pressure, all of which can result to fatty liver. Insulin also inhibits the breakdown of fat cells and even stimulates the creation of more body fat. This explains the weight gain. This coupled with the fact that as the body produces more fat, it starts experiencing what is referred to as leptin resistance (we will discuss leptin shortly). So with elevated levels of leptin hormone, your brain cannot tell when you have had enough so you will take more without even realizing it. This ultimately means you will be eating more calories resulting to more fat storage and the cycle continues.


So what causes insulin resistance in the first place? Well, the biggest contributor is foods high in sugars/fructose. That's why a sugar free diet is best for resetting your insulin.

## Meatless diet

Meatless diet controls estrogen.

Estrogen is a female sex hormone that deals with development and management of the female reproductive system. However, when in high quantities it is not good for you because it leads to bloating and water retention among other things that can make you gain weight. I am sure you are wondering how not eating meat can help you reset estrogen. Well, estrogen is often given to cattle to promote growth. If you eat meat, you will therefore tend to have higher level of estrogen than someone else who is a vegetarian due to the hormones in the meat. You have to maintain your estrogen and progesterone levels especially if you are a woman aged between 35 and 50 year since you will tend to have more estrogen already as compared to progesterone.

## Caffeine free diet

A coffee free diet resets your cortisol.

Caffeine triggers adrenal glands to produce more cortisol (the stress hormone) to initiate the "fight and flight" response. When you are constantly taking caffeinated drinks, you are constantly increasing your cortisol levels. This is not great because this hormone holds off burning of fat and preserves energy (the fight and flight response entails all that). This means that with high cortisol levels, you will be storing more fat rather than burning fat and this leads to weight gain.

Therefore, one of the effective ways of resetting cortisol hormone is not taking caffeine for some time.

# Fruit free diet

A fruitless diet resets your leptin.

Leptin or the satiety hormone is responsible for managing/regulating your balance of energy by inhibiting hunger when you have enough fat cells. Usually, the hormone will travel to the brain to send the signal that you have had enough. This means that if the hormone is not working, you will end up eating even when you have had enough. So where do fruits come in? Fruits contain sugar called fructose and having too much of it in your diet is linked to problems with insulin and leptin.

Fruits that we have currently are not the same as the ones that were available in the past. Although most diets will recommend fruits, most of the current fruits have been hybridized for sweetness, which means that they have more than 5 times the safe fructose levels.

Too much fructose in your body makes it hard for the liver to deal with it fast enough for use as fuel. Therefore, most of it ends up being converted to fat that is deposited in your belly and other parts of your body. When this happens, your level of leptin increases since leptin is released from fat cells and the more fat cells you have, the more leptin will be released. Over time, your body becomes resistant to leptin and it takes more production of leptin to send the signal that you have had enough, which is usually too late because you have eaten too much already.

Stay away from high fructose fruits and eat fruits like olives and avocadoes that are much better for your hormones.

## Toxin free

A toxin free diet will reset the testosterone.

Unfortunately, it is very difficult for us avoid the toxins because they have become a part of our lives. The food we eat is intoxicated right from the farm by fertilizers and pesticides not to forget the preservatives added before it is put in store shelves. The cleaning and the cosmetic products can also be toxic.

What you have to realize is that we are all exposed to plastic artificial chemicals in many different ways, which act as your endocrine disrupter. As a woman, it tends to raise your testosterone and as a man, it tends to lower your testosterone. This explains why girls today tend to enter the puberty stage so early and the male counterpart exhibits many female characteristics. The way to solving this imbalance is getting rid of the toxins.

If you reset your testosterone, you will find how easy it is to lose weight. This is especially because testosterone helps men build muscles, which ultimately boosts insulin sensitivity and when that happens, this makes it easier to lose weight, and achieve/maintain proper metabolic health just to mention a few of the benefits that come with testosterone. Actually, studies have proven that obesity results to reduced production of testosterone, which in turn is responsible for causing more fat storage. That's why men with reduced testosterone levels will gain weight easily especially when you couple the low testosterone levels with insulin resistance (a metabolic inability to handle carbohydrates). While losing weight in itself will boost your testosterone levels as a man, you have to lose weight first to get the benefits but if you are already in a vicious cycle, you have to break away from the cycle for this to work.

You can start by fighting toxins. And as you diet, you should insist on taking a diet rich in good fats (like olive oil and argan oil) and ample proteins (to help you build muscle, which ultimately helps you to boost testosterone production).

Note: These are not the only hormones whose imbalance has been linked with weight gain. Other hormones include growth hormone, which you can reset through a dairy free diet and grain free diet, which you can use to reset the thyroid- the thyroid is responsible for secreting several hormones like T3 and T4.

As you probably have noticed from the explanations, hormonal imbalance can have many effects; weight gain is just one of the many. So what are some of these other signs of hormonal imbalance?

*Other signs that you have a hormonal imbalance*

Apart from weight loss, the following signs are an indicator of hormone imbalance.

- Low libido

- Fatigue

- Cravings

- Digestive problems

- Constant fatigue

- Constant hunger

- Memory fog

- Persistent acne

- Sleep disorders

- Depression and mood swings

- Headache and migraines

- Weight gain

- Breast changes

- Hot flashes and nigh sweat

Note: While these are all signs that you have hormonal imbalance, they (the signs) could also signal some other underlying problems. Nonetheless, you need to take deliberate measures to fix the problem and this is through taking foods that will help you to reset your hormones. While the different hormones could be reset using different foods, approaching the matter holistically will definitely result to better effects. This is especially because if one hormone is not working well, then there is a high likelihood that another hormone is also not working well. In the next part of this book, I will show you some amazing recipes that you can follow to reset your hormones.

# Breakfast Recipes

## Goat Yogurt And Blueberry Smoothie

**Serves 1**

*Ingredients*

½ cup water

1 tablespoon chia seeds

½ cup blueberries, frozen

½ bananas, frozen

½ cup plain goat yogurt

1 serving whey protein isolate

*Instructions*

Combine all ingredients in a blender and blend on high speed until smooth.

# Cottage Cheese Oatmeal Pancakes

## Serves 2

*Ingredients*

1/2 cup teaspoon pure vanilla extract

1/4 teaspoon cinnamon

1/8 teaspoon baking powder

4 egg whites

1/2 cup low-fat cottage or ricotta cheese

1/2 cup quick cooking oats

1 tablespoon honey

*Instructions*

Combine all the ingredients in a blender and blend for a few seconds.

Spray a skillet with cooking spay then heat over medium heat then pour ¼ cup of the pancake mixture into the pan.

Cook until the edges appear set and bubbles appear on the top of the batter. Flip the pancake and cook until set in the center.

Repeat the same with the remaining batter.

# Tasty Omelette

## Serves 2

*Ingredients*

1 slice rye toast

2 teaspoons crumbled goat cheese

3 large egg whites

1 large omega-3 egg

½ cup sliced mushroom

A few slices red onion, chopped

¼ cup diced red bell pepper

¼ cup green bell pepper

1 tablespoon extra-virgin olive oil

*Instructions*

Over medium heat, heat olive oil in a small skillet and add red and green peppers, onions and mushrooms. Sauté until the vegetables soften.

Use a wire whisk to beat egg and egg whites in a small bowl until blended. Transfer the vegetables to a bowl and set aside once they are soft enough.

Into the same skillet, pour the egg mixture and cook for several minutes over medium heat until the eggs are set.

On one side of the cooked egg, evenly spread your vegetables and top with goat cheese. Use a spatula to fold the omelette in half over the vegetables. Enjoy with a piece of rye toast.

# Vanilla Green Milkshake

**Serves 1**

*Ingredients*

1 cup unsweetened coconut, hemp, or almond milk

6 pieces dinosaur kale with stem removed

½ avocado

2 scoops whey protein powder

2 tablespoons chia seeds soaked in unsweetened coconut, hemp, or almond milk for hours

A handful of ice cubes

*Instructions*

Add all the ingredients into a high-speed blender and blend on high. Serve and enjoy.

# Nutty Seedy Granola

## Serves 4

*Ingredients*

/2 teaspoon kosher salt

/2 teaspoon ground cinnamon

. teaspoon vanilla extract

3 tablespoons coconut oil

2 tablespoons water

egg lightly beaten

. cup unsweetened coconut

/2 cup sesame seeds

. cup raw or sprouted pumpkin seeds

. ½ cup raw almonds

. cup raw walnuts

*Instructions*

Preheat the oven to 300°F and line a baking sheet with parchment paper.

Add the walnuts, almonds, and pumpkin seeds to a high speed blender and pulse a few times to finely chop the nuts.

Whisk together egg whites with water in a large mixing bow until bubbly and slightly foamy.

Add the vanilla extract, cinnamon, and salt to the water/egg white combination then whisk them together. Into a mixing bowl, pour the chopped nut mixture along with the shredded coconut then stir until the mixture is coated.

Spread the granola evenly on the parchment-lined baking sheet and bake for 40 minutes.

Remove the granola from the oven and allow it to sit for 10 minutes, and then use a spatula to get under the granola and release the large clusters.

Place the granola in a sealable glass jar once it has cooled.

Serve over yogurt with fruit.

# Quinoa Porridge

## Serves 1

*Ingredients*

1 cup almond milk

1 cup quinoa

1 cup water

1 teaspoon vanilla extract

2 apples, grated with skin

1 tablespoon almonds, ground

½ teaspoon ground cinnamon

*Instructions*

Rinse the quinoa under running water.

Put the quinoa in a pot, add water and bring to a boil.

Reduce the heat and cook for 10 minutes or until soft. Make sure that the pot is covered.

Now add in cinnamon, vanilla, almonds, milk, apples and cinnamon and cook until nice and creamy. To make it creamier, you can add more milk.

Once done, serve with sliced banana.

# Apple Cinnamon Quinoa

## Serves 1

*Ingredients*

¼ cup dry quinoa

¼ cup water

2 tablespoons raisins

¼ cup almond milk

1 packet stevia

1 apple, chopped finely

¼ teaspoon cinnamon

1 tablespoon chia seeds

*Instructions*

Bring almond milk, quinoa and water to a boil in a pot.

Reduce the heat then simmer for around 5 minutes. Ensure that the pot is covered.

Add in the raisins, chia seeds, cinnamon, stevia, and apples and cook on low heat until all liquid is absorbed. This takes around 8-12 minutes.

# Lunch Recipes

## Maple Mustard Grilled Salmon

**Serves 4**

*Ingredients*

*For the glaze*

1/8 teaspoon pepper to taste

1/8 teaspoon sea salt to taste

1/2 teaspoon freshly chopped thyme

1 teaspoon apple cider vinegar

3 tablespoons whole grain mustard

1/3 cup maple syrup

*For the fish*

Pepper

Sea salt

Coconut oil or pure olive oil

4 (6-ounces) wild caught salmon fillets with skin on.

*Instructions*

Heat oil in a pan over medium heat then into the pan, place all the ingredients for making the glaze, and whisk them together. Heat until the liquid starts boiling then set aside.

Season the salmon fillets with salt and pepper and grill the side with the skin first for 3 minutes then flip to the other side and cook for an additional 3 minutes.

Remove the salmon from the pan and place on the plate. Brush each fillet with some of the glaze and serve.

# icken Coconut Curry Dish

## ves 2

*edients*

vn basmati rice

ı low fat coconut milk

2 tablespoons curry powder

2 boneless chicken breasts cut into strips

3 cloves of garlic, crushed

8 cups of spinach

1 large onion, chopped

2 tablespoons extra virgin oil

*Instructions*

Cook the brown basmati according to the package instructions.

Over medium heat, Sauté the chopped garlic and onions in olive oil in a large skillet then add chicken and curry powder. Cook on medium heat for 10 minutes while frequently stirring. Add the coconut milk and simmer for 20 more minutes.

Steam your spinach, drain it, then add to the chicken curry mix. Serve the mixture over the brown rice.

# Sweet And Crunchy Quinoa Salad

## Serves 2

*Ingredients*

4 scallions, sliced

½ teaspoon cinnamon

½ teaspoon ground cumin

¼ tablespoon ground black pepper

¼ teaspoon salt

4 teaspoons apple cider vinegar

1/3 cup pine nuts

3 tablespoons extra virgin olive oil, divided

1 medium sweet potato, peeled and cut into ½ inch cubes

1 cup quinoa, rinsed

*Instructions*

Preheat the oven to 400 °F

Place the quinoa in a small saucepan and add 2 cups of water. Bring to boil then simmer until the water has evaporated. Turn off the heat and let quinoa sit covered for at least one hour.

Place the sweet potato cubes into a roasting pan and toss with 1 ½ tablespoons of the olive oil. Bake for 25 minutes then set aside.

Place a pan over medium heat then add pine nuts and cook until lightly toasted.

Place the remaining 3 tablespoons of olive oil, cinnamon, cumin, pepper, salt and vinegar in a small bowl.

Once the quinoa is dry, break apart the seeds then place in a large bowl. Add half the vinaigrette and mix with the whisk. Add more to taste if you prefer it that way.

Add scallion, pine nuts, and sweet potatoes and mix gently.

Serve at room temperature.

# Tasty Broccoli Bacon Salad

## Serves 4

*Ingredients*

½ cup cherry tomatoes, halved

¼ cup sugar

2 tablespoons white vinegar

1 cup mayonnaise

8 ounces of sharp cheddar, chopped

½ cup raisins

½ cup chopped onions

6-8 slices cooked bacon, crumbled

1 small head of broccoli

*Instructions*

Chop broccoli into bite sized florets after removing the stems. Transfer this to a large bowl.

Add the bacon, tomatoes, cheese, cherries, and onion.

Combine vinegar, sugar, salt, pepper, and mayonnaise in another bowl then pour this into the large bowl with the broccoli mixture. Mix and enjoy.

# Refreshing Kale And Mango Salad

## Serves 4

*Ingredients*

¼ cup toasted sunflower seeds

1 ripe mango, peeled and diced

Black pepper to taste

Sea salt to taste

¼ cup extra virgin olive oil and more for drizzling on the salad

Juice of 1 lemon

1 bunch of kale

*Instructions*

Tear the leaves of the kale away from the stalk then tear the kale leaves into salad leaf size. Put the leaves into a bowl and drizzle with half of the lemon juice, a bit of oil then season with the salt.

Massage the lemon juice and oil into the kale using clean hands working it between your fingers until it is well coated in oil and has started to slightly wilt.

Combine the remaining half of lemon juice with olive oil and the pepper in a separate bowl. This will form your dressing.

Drizzle the dressing over the kale and toss to combine. Add the diced mango and toasted sunflower seeds. Serve.

*Hormone balancing ingredients in this include:*

Extra virgin olive oil

Sunflower seeds

Lemon, a citrus fruit

Kale

# Chicken And Lettuce Wraps

**Serves 2**

*Ingredients*

1 small head of lettuce

Salt and pepper to taste

¼ teaspoon low fat Greek yogurt

1 skinless and boneless chicken breast, cooked and diced

1 tablespoon finely chopped red onion

¼ cup diced cucumber

¼ cup diced red bell pepper

1 small green unpeeled and diced apple

*Instructions*

Combine all the ingredients in a bowl leaving out the lettuce. Chill for one hour then place the chicken mixture inside each lettuce leaf. Roll into cylinders and serve.

# Tuna With Vegetables

## Serves 4

*Ingredients*

2 carrots, sliced/julienned

2 quartered avocados

3 tablespoons sesame seeds

1 cup diced red bell pepper

2 cups chopped cabbage

16-20 ounces sushi grade tuna

¼ cup chopped cilantro

1 tablespoon lemon juice

*Instructions*

Mix all the ingredients except the tuna and sesame seeds in a bowl then set aside.

Coat tuna with sesame seeds then sear tuna in a hot pan with cooking spray.

Assemble each bowl by starting with vegetables with the some vegetables at the bottom, then tuna, avocado, and finally more vegetables.

# Dinner Recipes

## Summer Salad With Roasted Red Pepper Humus

*Serves 4*

*Ingredients*

/4 teaspoon salt and pepper

2 garlic cloves minced

. jalapeno, seeded and finely chopped

/4 cup extra virgin olive oil

/4 cup lime juice

. teaspoon grated lime or lemon

/4 cup freshly chopped cilantro

. avocado, diced

. red pepper, diced

. medium tomato, chopped

2 green onions, sliced thin

. (19 oz.) can of chickpeas, drained and rinsed

. (19 oz.) can of black beans, drained and rinsed.

*Instructions*

Into a large bowl, add cilantro, avocado, red pepper tomatoes, onions and the beans then toss to combine.

In a small separate bowl, mix the lime rind, pepper, salt jalapeno and oil juice and pour it over bean mixture then toss it all up. Serve with rice or tortillas.

# Cauliflower Salad

**Serves 4-6**

*Ingredients*

1/2 cup red onions, diced

3/4 cup diced celery

1/4 teaspoon black pepper

1/4 cup minced fresh dill

1 1/2 tablespoons brown mustard

3 tablespoon Thai canned coconut milk

2/3 cup grape seed oil Vegenaise

1/2 large cauliflower head

*Instructions*

Chop the cauliflower into florets and steam until tender, but not too tender.

Whisk the coconut milk, veganaise, pepper, dill, and mustard as the cauliflower is steaming.

Transfer the cauliflower into a large bowl once it is ready. Add onions and celery then toss the mixture gently.

Coat with the liquid mixture and toss gently again. Refrigerate until it is chilled then serve.

The hormone balancing ingredients here include onions and cauliflower.

# Turkey And Zucchini Lasagna

## Serves 6-8

*Ingredients*

1 can organic tomato sauce

1 teaspoon thyme

1 teaspoon sage

1 teaspoon rosemary

1 teaspoon dried basil

1 teaspoon oregano

4 organic egg whites

2 cloves of garlic minced

1 small yellow onion, finely chopped

1 teaspoon black pepper

2 teaspoons sea salt, divided

5 tablespoons olive oil, divided into half

1 teaspoon garlic powder

3 tablespoons coconut milk

2 cups chopped cauliflower

1 medium green bell pepper, finely chopped

1 medium red bell pepper, finely diced

1 (8 oz.) can tomato paste

1 pound lean ground organic turkey

2 tablespoons olive oil

6 large zucchinis

*Instructions*

Preheat oven to 350°F.

Slice zucchini lengthwise into very thin wide strips, and then sprinkle each strip with salt and set aside.

Heat 3 tablespoons olive oil in a large skillet over medium heat. Add onion and garlic then sauté until translucent. Stir in ground turkey and cook for approximately 4 minutes. Add all herbs and bell pepper and cook until the turkey is well browned.

Boil cauliflower until tender. Place cooked cauliflower pieces in a blender with the remaining 3 tablespoons of olive oil, coconut milk, garlic powder, salt, and pepper. Blend until creamy and smooth, adding more coconut milk if necessary.

Spray an 8 square inch baking dish with non-stick olive oil spray. Make the lining of the bottom of the baking dish with slices of zucchini. On top of zucchini, add a thin layer of turkey mixture on. Add a layer of tomato sauce then ¼ inch thick layer of cauliflower that is blended to cover this layer.

Repeat the layering of cauliflower, tomato sauce, meat and zucchini, as many layers as you want. Make an even layer of frothy egg on top of lasagna after beating. Bake at 350 degrees for about 25 minutes or until the eggs are set.

Serve and enjoy.

# Roasted Shallot, Squash, And Green Bean Salad

## Serves 4

*Ingredients*

1 large bunch of watercress, chopped

½ teaspoon garlic, minced

1 ¼ teaspoons rosemary, finely chopped

1 ½ tablespoons apple cider vinegar

1 cup of grapes

Pure olive oil and extra virgin oil

4 large shallots peeled and quartered lengthwise

2 zucchini, sliced

1 butter squash

6 oz. green beans, trimmed

*Instructions*

Preheat the oven to 425 F.

Peel the neck of the squash and slice the entire neck into ½-inch wheels to obtain 8 wheels.

In a large bowl, toss zucchini, shallots and squash with about 2 tablespoons of olive oil. Season with salt and pepper and arrange on a baking sheet.

n the same bowl with squash, toss the grapes and green beans to coat with the remaining oil. Arrange the grapes and green beans on the same baking sheet but separate a little bit from the other vegetables for easy removal.

Roast the vegetables for 8 minutes until the green beans are crisp and the grapes are heated through. Remove the green beans and grapes to a separate plate and set aside.

Continue to roast the squash and shallots for about 20 minutes more.

In a small bowl, whisk together 2 ½ tablespoons of oil, garlic, vinegar and rosemary. Season with salt and pepper while the squash is roasting.

Serve by laying each plate with a bit of watercress and the grapes and vegetables then drizzle with the dressing.

# Avocado Salad

## Serves 2

*Ingredients*

Handful of sunflower seeds

Sea salt to taste

½ tomato, diced

2 cloves of garlic, minced

Extra virgin olive oil

Juice of ½ a lemon

2 avocadoes

*Instructions*

Cut the avocadoes into quarters, seed them, remove the skin then chop the quarters into smaller pieces.

Combine the chopped avocado with sea salt, tomato, garlic, and lemon juice in a bowl. Spoon the mixture back into a bowl and sprinkle with raw or toasted sunflower seeds.

Serve and enjoy.

# Tahini Roasted Cauliflower

## Serves 4

*Ingredients*

Salt and pepper to taste

½ teaspoon garlic powder

¼ teaspoon cumin

Zest and juice of 1 lemon

1 cup tahini

1 head of cauliflower

*Instructions*

Preheat oven to 400°F

Wash cauliflower and trim off all leaves and cut the bottom.

Mix tahini, cumin, juice, lemon zest, pepper salt and garlic powder in a small bowl.

Line a baking sheet with foil or parchment pepper. Drizzle olive oil or grape seed oil on the baking sheet so that the cauliflower will not stick.

Massage tahini mixture over cauliflower.

Roast in oven until it becomes fork tender.

Serve and enjoy.

# Grilled Veggies With Quinoa

## Serves 4

*Ingredients*

### Quinoa

½ red bell pepper, seeded and finely diced

2 garlic cloves minced

2 shallots, minced

1½ tablespoons extra-virgin olive oil

2cups quinoa, soaked for 1 hour and rinsed

Salt and pepper to taste

### Veggies

¼ teaspoon fresh thyme

2 tablespoons extra virgin olive oil

1 large avocado, halved

1 medium zucchini, halved lengthwise

½ lb. asparagus, trimmed

1 large tomato cut in half

### Garnish

4 large leaves fresh basil, rolled then cut into strips

Toasted walnuts

¾ cup black olives

A bed of fresh mixed greens

## Dressing

1½ tablespoons lemon juice

1½ tablespoons balsamic vinegar

3½ tablespoons extra virgin oil

Salt and pepper to taste

*Instructions*

In a large saucepan, place the quinoa and cover slightly with water. Cook for fifteen minutes then remove and put in a large bowl to cool.

Heat oil in a skillet over medium heat and sauté the shallots, red pepper, and garlic until soft. Season with salt and pepper to taste then transfer to the quinoa and mix well.

Heat the grill pan to medium. Place the vegies on a baking sheet and brush well with oil. Grill the vegies for about 5 minutes, place the grilled vegies on a cutting board then add thyme and chopped vegetables into bite size pieces.

Place a bed of greens on a large platter, top with quinoa, place the vegies on the quinoa, and add the garnish on top.

Whisk the lemon, vinegar, and olive oil together and pour over the salad. Season with salt and fresh black pepper to taste

Serve and enjoy.

# Soup Recipes

## Kale And Bean Soup

**Serves 6**

*Ingredients*

1 lemon juiced and zested

1 (14.5 ounce) can of drained and rinsed cannellini beans

2 tablespoons rosemary, chopped

14.5 ounce can Italian-style diced tomatoes

4 cups kale, packed and chopped

1 (32 ounce) box low-sodium vegetable broth

4 large garlic cloves

2 large carrots, peeled and sliced

1 cup yellow onion, diced

2 tablespoons extra-virgin oil

*Instructions*

Heat olive oil in a large sized saucepan over medium heat. Add onion and cook for 3 minutes. Add carrots and cook for an additional 3 minutes. Add garlic and cook for 2 minutes longer.

Add broth, sea salt, tomatoes, beans, kale, and rosemary and cover then Cook for 5 minutes.

Add lemon zest and juice, stir then serve hot

# Asparagus, Fennel And Dill Soup

**Serves 7**

*Ingredients*

Freshly ground black pepper to taste

1 lemon, zested

3 tablespoons fresh lemon juice

3 cups light vegetable broth

½ cup fresh mint leaves, loosely packed

½ cup fresh dill, loosely packed

2 tablespoons olive oil

2 large leeks

3 tablespoons brown rice

1 ½ teaspoons sea salt

4 cups water

1 bunch green onions, sliced

10 oz. asparagus, sliced

10 oz. fennel bulbs, chopped

10 oz. sugars snap peas, stringed and coarsely chopped

*Instructions*

Wash all the vegetables and put them in a large pot with water, rice, and 1 tablespoon salt. Cover the pot and simmer for about 30 minutes.

Sauté the chopped green onions in olive oil over medium heat with a pinch of salt. Stir often until they become translucent.

Add the mint, dill, cooked onions, and broth to the vegetables.

Let the soup simmer for a few minutes then remove from heat and let it cool for a while.

Pour the soup in a blender and puree in a blender until smooth.

Return it to the pot and add sea salt, pepper and lemon juice to taste. Bring the soup back to a simmer before you serve.

Drizzle some fruity olive oil on top of each serving and enjoy.

# Detox Broth

**Serves 4**

*Ingredients*

½ teaspoon turmeric powder

Juice of one lemon

1 tablespoon fresh herbs such as parsley

2 tablespoons fresh ginger root, minced

2 cups of a about 3 vegetables such as kale, green beans, roughly chopped

4 cups bone broth from an organic chicken

Sea salt to taste

*Instructions*

Place chopped vegetables in a stockpot and cover with bone broth. Bring to boil and then simmer for 40 minutes. Add lemon juice, herbs, and turmeric powder.

Serve and enjoy.

# Cauliflower Soup

## Serves 4

*Ingredients*

Salt and pepper to taste

2 tablespoons tahini

4 cups organic chicken broth

1 russet potato, cut into 1 inch cubes

1 head cauliflower, cut into florets

1 clove garlic, minced

1 medium onion, coarsely chopped

1 tablespoon olive oil

Silvered almonds, to garnish

*Instructions*

Heat oil in a large pot over medium heat and sauté garlic and onions until the onions are translucent.

Add cauliflower and potato and continue cooking for about 3 minutes. Add chicken broth and bring to boil, reduce the heat and simmer until the potato is fork-tender.

Add tahini then using an immersion blender, blend the soup until it is smooth and velvety.

Toast the almonds.

60

Season the soup with pepper and salt and garnish with almonds.

# Chicken Broth

## Yields: 4 quarts of broth

*Ingredients*

1 bunch parsley

3 celery sticks, coarsely chopped

2 carrots, peeled and coarsely chopped

1 large onion, coarsely chopped

2 tablespoons of apple cider vinegar

3 liters of cold filtered water

Head from one chicken, optional

1 organic chicken

Feet from the chicken

Gizzards from 1 chicken

*Instructions*

Cut the chicken into several pieces after chopping off the head, wings, and neck.

Put the chicken pieces, vinegar and water and all the vegetables except for parsley in steel pot.

Let it stand for 30 minutes before you bring it to boil. Cover the pot and then reduce the heat to simmer.

Simmer for 12 hours on low heat and remember to add parsley a few minutes before finishing cooking.

Remove the large chicken pieces and let them cool then remove the flesh from the carcass.

Strain the stock into a large bowl and let it cool in the fridge until the fat rises to the top and congeals.

Skim off the fat and reserve the stock in covered glass containers. Freeze some of the stock for maximum freshness

# Lentil Soup

**Serves 4**

*Ingredients*

2 tablespoons tomato paste

4 cups vegetable stock

1 cup dry red lentils

1 teaspoon sea salt

1 teaspoon cinnamon

1 tablespoon curry powder

1 inch piece fresh ginger root, peeled and minced

4 cloves garlic, minced

1 large onion, chopped

1 sweet potato, peeled and diced

2 tablespoons extra-virgin oil

*Instructions*

Over medium heat, heat olive oil in a large saucepan then add onions, sweet potato, ginger, garlic and cook until vegetables are softened.

Stir in the cinnamon, sea salt, and curry powder and cook for a few more minutes.

Add the vegetable stock, lentils, and tomato paste and mix well. Bring to a gentle boil and reduce the heat, cover it then simmer for 30 minutes until lentils are cooked.

Remove from the heat and serve.

# White Beans And Swiss Chard Soup

## Serves 4

*Ingredients*

Salt and pepper to taste

30 ounces of Northern beans, drained and rinsed

4 cups chopped Swiss chard with stems removed

6 cups of chicken broth, low-sodium

2 garlic cloves, minced

1 cup chopped onions

1 (1-pound) package of turkey or chicken sausage with the casings removed

*Instructions*

Brown the sausage, garlic and onions in a large pot over medium heat until the sausage is cooked through and crumbly. Add in the broth, Swiss chard and beans then stir.

Season with salt and pepper to taste then bring the pot to boil. Reduce the heat and simmer covered for about 20 minutes or until the Swiss chard is wilted and tender.

Serve immediately alone or with a small side salad.

# Sweet Creamy Soup

## Serves 4-6

*Ingredients*

1 (8-ounce) organic sprouted tofu cut into small cubes

1 cup sprouted adzuki beans

2 stalks, diced

1 white or yellow onion, diced

1 sweet potato, peeled and cubed

4-6 cups vegetable stock or organic chicken stock

Fermented shoyu to taste

Savory herbs to taste

Baby greens to garnish

*Instructions*

Place the beans, sweet potato, celery, onions and stock in a large pot. Bring this to a boil then lower the heat and simmer for 25 minutes or until the beans are cooked.

Now add in the herbs and tofu, stir and cook for five minutes.

Allow the soup to cool slightly then process in blender in batches until smooth and creamy then add shoyu and garnish with some baby greens.

# Conclusion

We have come to the end of the book. Thank you for reading and congratulations for reading until the end.

As I had earlier mentioned, sometimes, losing weight is not just about creating a caloric deficit. It is also about resetting hormones that could be actually sabotaging your goals to lose weight. Use everything you've learned in this book to make an informed decision regarding your diet.

If you found the book valuable, can you recommend it to others? One way to do that is to post a review on Amazon.

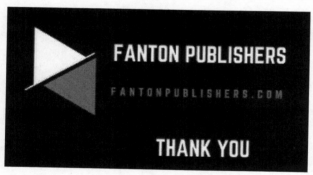

# Do You Like My Book & Approach To Publishing?

If you like my writing and style and would love the ease of learning literally everything you can get your hands on from Fantonpublishers.com, I'd really need you to do me either of the following favors.

# 6 Things

I'll be honest; publishing books on what I learn in my line of work gives me satisfaction. But the biggest satisfaction that I can get as an author is knowing that I am influencing people's lives positively through the content I publish. Greater joy even comes from knowing that customers appreciate the great content that they have read in every book through giving feedback, subscribing to my newsletter, sending emails to tell me how transformative the content they read is, following me on social media and buying several of my books. That's why I am always seeking to engage my readers at a personal level to know them and for them to know me, not just as an author but as a person because we all want to belong. That's why I strive to use different channels to engage my readers so that I can ultimately build a cordial relationship with them for our mutual success i.e. I succeed as an author while at the same time my readers learn stuff that takes days and sometimes weeks to write, edit, format and publish in a matter of hours.

To build this relationship, I'd really appreciate if you could do any or all the following:

# 1: First, I'd Love It If You Leave a Review of This Book on Amazon.

Let me be honest; reviews play a monumental role in determining whether customers purchase different products online. From the thousands of other books that are on Amazon about the topic, you chose to read this one. I am grateful for that. I may not know why you read my book, especially until the end considering the fact that most readers don't read until the end. Perhaps you purchased this book after reading some of the reviews and were glued with reading the book because it was educative and engaging. Even if you didn't read it because of the positive reviews, perhaps you can make the next customer's purchasing decision a lot easier by posting a review of this book on Amazon!

I'd love it if you did that, as this would help me spread word out about my books and publishing business. The more the readers, the bigger a community we build and we all benefit! If you could leave your honest review of this book on Amazon, I'd be forever grateful (well, I am already grateful to you for purchasing the book and reading it until the end- I don't' take that for granted!). Please Leave a Review of This Book on Amazon.

## 2: Check Out My Other Books

As I stated earlier, my biggest joy in all this is building an audience that loves my approach to publishing and the amazing content I publish. I know every author has his/her style. Mine is publishing what I learn to readers out there so that they can learn what is trending, what other readers are also searching for in the nonfiction world and much more. As such, if you read the other books I have published, you will undoubtedly know a lot more than the average person on a diverse range of issues. And as you well know, knowledge is power- and the biggest investment that you can ever have on your life!

**PS:** If you want me to filter everything for you to include only Ketogenic diet books, you can subscribe to my newsletter and I will send you a list of all my Ketogenic diet books along with other useful content that I come across to ensure you succeed while at it http://bit.ly/2Cketodietfanton.

# 3: Let's Get In Touch

Let's get closer than just leaving reviews and buying my other books. Reach out to me through email, like or follow me on social media and let's interact. You will perhaps get to know stuff about me that will change your life in a way. As we interact, we will also influence each other in a way. I' definitely would love to learn something from you as we get to know each other.

**Antony**

**Website**: http://www.fantonpublishers.com/

**Email:** Support@fantonpublishers.com

**Twitter**: https://twitter.com/FantonPublisher

**Facebook** **Page:**
https://www.facebook.com/Fantonpublisher/

**My Ketogenic Diet Books Page:**
**https://www.facebook.com/pg/Fast-Keto-Meals-336338180266944**

**Private Facebook Group For Readers:**
https://www.facebook.com/groups/FantonPublishers/

**Pinterest**: https://www.pinterest.com/fantonpublisher/

## 4: Grab Some Freebies On Your Way Out; Giving Is Receiving, Right?

I gave you 2 freebies at the start of the book, one on general life transformation and one about the Ketogenic diet. You are free to choose either or both!

**Ketogenic Diet Freebie**: http://bit.ly/2fantonpubketo

**5 Pillar Life Transformation Checklist**: http://bit.ly/2fantonfreebie

## 5: Suggest Topics That You'd Love Me To Cover To Increase Your Knowledge Bank. As I stated, I love feedback; any type of feedback- positive or negative. As such, make sure to reach out. I am looking forward to seeing your suggestions and insights on the topic. You could even suggest improvements to this book. Simply send me a message on Support@fantonpublishers.com. As a publisher, I strive to publish content that my readers are

actively looking for. Therefore, your input is highly important.

## 6: <u>Subscribe To My Newsletter</u> To Know When I Publish New Books.

I already mentioned this earlier; I love to connect with my readers. This is just another avenue for me to connect to you. As such, if you would love to know whenever I publish new books and blog posts, subscribe to my newsletter at http://bit.ly/2fantonpubnewbooks. You will be the first to know whenever I have fresh content!

rfort the titles on Amazon.

### General Weight Loss Books

The books in this category will help you lose weight irrespective of the approach you are using i.e. dieting or workout. I recommend you have them even if you are on specific diets or using specific workouts for weight loss.

**Binge Eating: Binge Eating Disorder Cure: Easy To Follow Tips For Eating Only What Your Body Needs**

**Lose Weight: Lose Weight Fast Naturally: How to Lose Weight Fast Without Having To Become a Gym Rat or Dieting Like a Maniac**

**Lose Weight: Lose Weight Permanently: Effective Strategies on How to Lose Weight Easily and Permanently**

**Get updates when we publish any book about weight loss: http://bit.ly/2fantonweightlossbooks**

74

# Weight Loss Books On Specific Diets

# Ketogenic Diet Books

KETOGENIC DIET: Keto Diet Made Easy: Beginners Guide on How to Burn Fat Fast With the Keto Diet (Including 100+ Recipes That You Can Prepare Within 20 Minutes)- New Edition

KETOGENIC DIET: Ketogenic Diet Recipes That You Can Prepare Using 7 Ingredients and Less in Less Than 30 Minutes

Ketogenic Diet: With A Sustainable Twist: Lose Weight Rapidly With Ketogenic Diet Recipes You Can Make Within 25 Minutes

Ketogenic Diet: Keto Diet Breakfast Recipes

Get updates when we publish any book on the Ketogenic diet: http://bit.ly/2fantonpubketo

# Intermittent Fasting Books

Intermittent Fasting: A Complete Beginners Guide to Intermittent Fasting For Weight Loss, Increased Energy, and A Healthy Life

Get updates when we publish any book on intermittent fasting: http://bit.ly/2fantonbooksIF

# Any Other Diet

Hormone Reset Diet: 31 Hormone Reset Diet Recipes to Hormone Balance, FAST Weight Loss, Lower Stress, Better Immune System, and Faster Metabolism

Get updates when we publish any book on any other diet that will help you to lose weight and keep it off: http://bit.ly/2fantonsdietbooks

## Relationships Books

Wedding: Budget Wedding: Wedding Planning On The Cheap (Master How To Plan A Dream Wedding On Budget)

How To Get Your Ex Back: Step By Step Formula On How To Get Your Ex Back And Keep Him/her For Good

SEX POSITIONS: Sex: Unleash The Tiger In You Using These 90-Day Sex Positions With Pictures

Money Problems: How To Solve Relationship Money Problems: Save Your Marriage By Learning How To Fix All Your Money Problems And Save Your Relationship

Family Communication: A Simple Powerful Communication Strategy to Transform Your Relationship with Your Kids and Enjoy Being a Parent Again

Get updates when we publish any book that will help you improve on your personal and professional relationships: http://bit.ly/2fantonsrelations

# Personal Development

Body Language: Master Body Language: A Practical Guide to Understanding Nonverbal Communication and Improving Your Relationships

Subconscious Mind: Tame, Reprogram & Control Your Subconscious Mind To Transform Your Life

Emotional Intelligence: The Mindfulness Guide To Mastering Your Emotions, Getting Ahead And Improving Your Life

Habits: The Habit Blueprint: 15 Simple Steps to Transform Your Life and Create Lasting Change without Feeling Overwhelmed and Frustrated

Get updates when we publish any book that will help you become a better person by boosting your productivity, achieving more of your goals, beating procrastination, breaking bad habits, forming new habits, beat stress, building your self-esteem and confidence and much more: http://bit.ly/2fantonpubpersonaldevl

# Personal Finance & Investing Books

Real Estate: Rental Property Investment Guide: How To Buy & Manage Rental Property For Profits

MONEY: Make Money Online: 150+ Real Ways to Make Real Money Online (Plus 50 Bonus Tips to Guarantee Your Success)

Money: How To Make Money Online: Make Money Online In 101 Ways

Get updates when we publish any book that will help you up your game in personal finance and investing: http://bit.ly/2fantonpersfinbooks

## Health & Fitness Books

PMS CURE: Easy To Follow Home Remedies For PMS & PMDD

Testosterone: How to Boost Your Testosterone Levels in 15 Different Ways Naturally

Hair Loss: How to Stop Hair Loss: Actionable Steps to Stop Hair Loss (Hair Loss Cure, Hair Care, Natural Hair Loss Cures)

Hashimoto's: Hashimoto's Cookbook: Eliminate Toxins and Restore Thyroid Health through Diet In 1 Month

Stress: The Psychology of Managing Pressure: Practical Strategies to turn Pressure into Positive Energy (5 Key Stress Techniques for Stress, Anxiety, and Depression Relief)

Get updates when we publish any book that will help you up your game in health and fitness: http://bit.ly/2fantonhealthnfit

# Book Summaries

This category will feature summaries of some of your favorite books, written in a manner you can easily digest and follow:

**Summary: The Millionaire Next Door: The Surprising Secrets of America's Wealthy**

**Summary: The Plant Paradox: The Hidden Dangers In "Healthy" Foods That Cause Disease And Weight Gain**

**Get updates whenever we publish new book summaries:** http://bit.ly/2fantons

# All The Other Niches

This category of books includes anything that we cannot realistically fit in the categories above. As always, if you want just about anything you can get to read, this is the category for you!

## Travel Books

**Kenya: Travel Guide: The Traveler's Guide to Make The Most Out of Your Trip to Kenya (Kenya Tourists Guide)**

## Dog Training

Dog Tricks: 15 Tricks You Must Teach Your Dog before Anything Else

## World Issues Books

ISIS/ISIL: The Rise and Rise of the Islamic State: A Comprehensive Guide on ISIS & ISIL

**Get notifications when we publish books on anything else above from the niches I mentioned above:** http://bit.ly/2fantonpubnewbooks

# See You On The Other Side!

See, I publish books on just about any topic imaginable!

If you have any suggestions on topics you would want me to cover, feel free to get in touch:

**Website**: http://www.fantonpublishers.com/

**Email:** Support@fantonpublishers.com

**Twitter**: https://twitter.com/FantonPublisher

**My Ketogenic Diet Books Page:** https://www.facebook.com/pg/Fast-Keto-Meals-336338180266944

**Facebook** **Page**: https://www.facebook.com/Fantonpublisher/

**Private Facebook Group For Readers:** https://www.facebook.com/groups/FantonPublishers/

**Pinterest**: https://www.pinterest.com/fantonpublisher/

PS: You can subscribe to my mailing list to know when I publish new books:

Hey! This is not the entire list! You can check an updated list of all my books on:

**My Author Central**: amazon.com/author/fantonpublishers

**My Website**: http://www.fantonpublishers.com

# Stay With Me On My Journey To Making Passive Income Online

I have to admit; my writing business makes several six figures a year in profits (after paying ourselves salaries). Until recently, I didn't realize just how hard we worked to build this business to what it has become so far.

However, while it is profitable and I want to do it in the long term, I understand its limitations. I know I cannot have an endless number of writers at a time especially if we are to continue delivering high quality products to our customers and readers consistently.

That's why I have recently started getting more serious with self-publishing to help me build a passive income business i.e. income that is not pegged on the number of writers and hours that we put to develop our products.

Thanks to my vast experience and dedication to get things done, I am committed to building a six figure passive income publishing business.

To make sure you are part of this journey, I am inviting you to subscribe to our newsletter (http://bit.ly/2fanton6figprogress) to know my progress as far as passive income generation is concerned. That's not all; if making passive income, just like me, is something you'd love to venture into, you can follow my 'tell it all' blog, which I explain everything I have done to promote every book and how the results are turning out with figures and images.

My goal is to make sure that while I add value to my audience through the different topics that I publish about to solve various problems for instance, I also add massive value to readers in ways that go beyond just one book. Subscribe to our newsletter to know when I publish new books, how I did market research, how I make money with the books and much, much more.

You can even ask questions on anything you want me to answer regarding publishing and everything else related to the topics of discussion.

**Antony**

**Website**: http://www.fantonpublishers.com/

**Email:** Support@fantonpublishers.com

**Twitter**: https://twitter.com/FantonPublisher

**Facebook** **Page:** https://www.facebook.com/Fantonpublisher/

**My Ketogenic Diet Books Page: https://www.facebook.com/pg/Fast-Keto-Meals-336338180266944**

**Private Facebook Group For Readers:** https://www.facebook.com/groups/FantonPublishers/

**Pinterest**: https://www.pinterest.com/fantonpublisher/

I look forward to hearing from you!

# PSS: Let Me Also Help You Save Some Money!

If you are a heavy reader, have you considered subscribing to Kindle Unlimited? You can read this and millions of other books for just $9.99 a month)! You can check it out by searching for Kindle Unlimited on Amazon!

Made in the USA
Lexington, KY
18 February 2019